universe we exist in and are a part of. The atoms that are the energy and power of all that is are what we are made up of too, what we are connected with and that power lays deep in us, just waiting to be used for the greater good, for the evolving of who we are to our true potential and purpose, to great love and unlimited achievement as a united people. This is my dream, this is something beautiful we can bring to reality.

THE RIGHTS OF THE MANY

It is damn heartbreaking that so many in this day and age are still made to feel like lesser human beings. Why should someone be treated worse because they were born a woman or a different color or love someone of the same gender. How dare people make others feel worse because of the way they were born. What gives them the right to make the lives of anyone harder because of how they were born? It is horrible that love when given to someone of the same gender is treated with disgust and derision when it is still love, the most purest thing there is. Love is love, no matter the gender. It is the sweetest, most beautiful feeling there is and for it to be treated as something bad or wrong is what's wrong. What is just as bad is for someone to be treated with less rights because they were born a different color or born a woman, like what the hell? We are all humans, born into this world as humans and shall perish from this earth as humans. Women carry us in their wombs, give birth to us, and in most cases, nurture us and love us, in so many cases on their own, no matter how hard it gets or what they have to sacrifice from their lives. They are the most beautiful humans, the ones that give birth to life. Think about that. They carry life in them and give birth to it from their very own bodies, enduring immense pain in the process so a new life can come into this world. Why should they get paid less or treated as less, given less power when it is both sexes that make all possible, when they can do exactly what men can do. I wish I could be half the parent that my mother was to me and my sister when she had to do it alone when we were kids. The strength, determination and reliance she showed is still an inspiration to me today and I will never forget just how powerful it made me realize women are when I was growing up in a time when women still served the men. My mother will always be my hero for what she did and who she is, someone so full of love and kindness and such a genuine caring heart. A beautiful soul. Now, on the subject of racism. Why the heck is it that in places like Australia and America where so many of the population are and descend from European white immigrates, we think immigrates of a different skin color don't deserve to be in the countries we live in? Why shouldn't they have equal rights if they are willing to work and contribute? Why do white people go on about 'oh, they're taking all our jobs!?' when nothing is said about white immigrates coming over and working and living? I understand the fear of terrorists coming in but that only accounts for a small amount of countries in the world, a few places where terrorism grows strong. It does not give anyone the right to say someone else doesn't belong or doesn't deserve the same rights or equal opportunity because of their skin color. I think people that have done all they could, fought tooth and nail for a better life for themselves and their families in a better country than where they came from should be given so much respect for that and not treated like shit or made to fear for the safety and lives of them and their family, their children. The continued mistreatment of people born in our countries who have different colored skin is just as shocking. What possible reason could there be to treat them worse like lesser people except for small minded and weak people needing to make themselves feel bigger or more important. It's time for human rights to take another big step forward and everyone embrace equality for all that it stands for. This includes no more using the n word for black people, no more using the f word for gays or the b word for women. Let's make a difference and things equal and fair for all of the above because it is the right thing to do. Humanity means all of us. We all stand together on this earth, birth to death so let's do it united as equals to make us stronger as a united people. Together we can forge through the hardest of times and accomplish anything. With great love and understanding, equality among all, there is nothing we can't achieve as the power of us all walking this earth together will be incredible and unstoppable. Let's make the change that is needed. Let us join together, arm in arm, hand in hand, all brothers and sisters and make a better tomorrow. We can do it. Oh yes we can!

EVOLVING AS A SOCIETY TOWARDS UTOPIA

What do you think of when you imagine Utopia? Somewhere where suffering has been reduced to a minimum? Somewhere full of love? A society with no war, famine, disease? I imagine all those things but some of the main things I think a Utopian society would have are love, kindness, positivity, understanding and acceptance by and for all. I think in some ways we have been evolving towards it. As tolerance and pc behavior has become more of the norm, it shows we are evolving in the right way towards a bliss filled utopia. Those that argue against being pc have their arguments which are fair enough from their point of view and they can't be blamed but it is the mindset of the past and if we truly want to reach a utopian future, we need to move away from old mindsets. When people talk down about pc behavior with sayings like 'toughen up' n 'don't be so weak' 'stop being so butthurt' and they complain about people getting feelings hurt, they themselves are showing they are still stuck in the old mindset from times where people didn't talk about feelings, didn't show they were hurt. Times where LGBT people, people with different colored skin and women were treated as not good enough, had horrible things done to them which were accepted as the norm and okay. We have begun to slowly move away from that type of behavior and mindset, well a lot of us anyway which is a massive step towards evolution as a society and becoming a utopia. A utopia where everyone can feel safe in being who they are, who they were born as instead of living their lives feeling inferior, living like a second even third class citizen. I get why people can feel so frustrated about a fuss being made about not hurting people's feelings, people being sensitive. I worked as a rooftiler for years and also grew up in Australia so there was a lot of name calling 'hanging shit' as we call it and it was just the norm, mostly didn't mean anything so I do understand why the old mindset people find it so infuriating and nonsense. But having said that, for us to reach utopia, to truly find that pure level of evolved society, there shouldn't have to be people putting up with being degraded in any way. As much as people laugh it off when it is among mates and co-workers, there are a million others in the world whom are hurt, mind messed with and love of self-injured. I understand where people are coming from when they rage against the 'pussying down of society' and the thought that everyone should be strong and learn to harden up, learn how to take things better instead of getting hurt but that is where we came from as a society, not where we are going. That is how it was when we lived in darker times, a more primitive age in the world and now we need to keep moving forward towards a time where love and kindness is the main trait, not being hard or tough. This doesn't mean people still can't be tough and strong or that we will all turn to weaklings, it just means we grow to a point where feelings are respected, good energy is let flow instead of negativity and hate. Strength will always be needed, just not nastiness. I ache to be a part of this dream I dream, this Utopia where love and pure good energy is the way of society. I may be called a fool for this as great change generally takes a long time but we can bring utopia closer quicker. We can have it in our time if we keep moving forward with open hearts and understanding, love and kindness. We must let go of stale mindsets that hold us as a society back so utopia can come to us with greater haste. Slaves were freed because it was the right thing to do in the name of humanity and equality but so many didn't think so yet there is still unfair and racist treatment by so many. Gay people are allowed to marry in more and more places because it is their basic human right to be able to do so but people still say it goes against god and even people that support the love of those in the LGBT community say they still shouldn't be allowed to marry. Women operate in the world just as men do for the most part these days, do the same jobs, get the same education but are still paid less in many areas, still treated as inferior by many. Bullying of so many people still causes so many suicides, so many lost lives that could have been saved if kindness was more ingrained in the mindset of society. So many beautiful souls, dead forever. So many wounded hearts lost from the world as we know it. It breaks my heart. We have come such a far way and there is much work to be done but only so much before we reach the beginnings of a utopia like time. With great, wide spread communication, understanding, patience and love we can spark an even bigger change to sweep through society. What kind of world do we want our kids and their generation and the next generation to grow into? Sure some will say they want their kids to be tough and not emotionally weak or so sensitive but a better way to look at it would be would you rather your child be caring and understanding of others, to give good energy and emotional strength to others or be someone that breaks others down, doesn't care if feelings are hurt and spread bad and hurtful energy into the world? We are an amazing people, humanity has so much love and kindness in it already. We are filled with limitless potential from the power of the world and

BULLYING

What to do about a problem like bullying? The answer becomes more difficult when so many think it is a valuable part of life that toughens up kids and yes, it may toughen up some but for most others, the ones that can't handle it, it can ruin a life, cause lasting mental scars, social issues and also push people to suicide. Whilst still young and many years later when problems stemming from the original bullying have piled up and become too much too handle. Of course there is two sides of bullying, the victims and the attackers and I will try and speak on both sides, try to show understanding. To begin with, I was bullied for so very many years through primary and high school which has caused me untold social anxieties, self-esteem issues, trouble with making friends and so much more. So on the victim side, as I have touched on, it might only seem like a bit of teasing but that's not what it feels like, especially when one is copping it from so many with nobody on one's side and each time it sinks further and further into heart and mind until confidence is stripped to nothing, self-esteem is drained and happiness gets replaced with depression, despair, loneliness, anger and so many thoughts and feelings that just weighs one's soul down with such heavy weight that some never recover. It's easy to say just laugh it off or laugh at self so they don't or stand up for self so they don't see you as easy target and leave you alone but it isn't so easy to do, especially when one's confidence has already been worn down. I think that every teacher should have at least some level of qualification in counselling so there is more help available to any students going through problems. Even then, so many kids going through it find they can't talk to anyone about it or that when they do they aren't listened to properly or understood with how much of a problem it actually is for them.

The issues that can come from being bullied can be so hard for a young person to explain as well, the complicated down feelings that come from it. Now, on the other side of the coin. People that bully think it is just messing around, a bit of teasing and means nothing, most of the time completely unaware of the damage they could be doing. So many do it just to be on the majority side of the crowds, to fit in. Others do it to feel better about themselves if they are having issues. Some do it because it is what they get off others, a lot of the time because they cop similar treatment or worse in their own home from family members and it just becomes a way of life, something given, learned and kept going. With the ones that are doing it just to fit in and go along with what others are doing, look cool, be popular, not picked on themselves, greater understanding can be grown about how damaging it can be and they can learn. The ones that do know just how much damage they are doing and bully even worse because of it are people I don't know what to say about. Well I don't have anything nice or understanding to say on their behalf as anyone that knowingly pushes someone towards suicide and depression disgusts me and makes me so angry. Now when it is someone that is copping it at home, going through the same thing and worse themselves and find themselves passing the bad treatment on, it makes it so tricky for schools to handle as nobody deserves to go through it and the last thing schools want is a kid who does it cause of what goes on at home, getting in trouble and copping it even worse at home. There can be counselling at school provided for these bullies whom come from being bullied at home but that only does so much and it doesn't stop the treatment or cycle of abuse at home. Sure there would be some parents that would listen and learn but most would not take it well, someone telling them how to raise their child and in the case of it being one of the simpler forms of bullying at home, just words here and there, would calling child services really be the right option, breaking up a family because of words? There would have to be something done, something said to break the cycle though. People are losing who they are, their light, their entire personalities and even taking their own lives because of bullying and it has to end. I know some will say kids just need to learn how to handle it but like I said before, by the time they realize something needs to be done, they have already lost their confidence and strength and damage sets in so deep and fast with children, even if it goes unnoticed for a long time. Yes, learning to laugh at oneself so others won't and learning how to stand up for self so you don't get picked on is important and can help so many and should be taught by parents as much as possible but this article is about the ones that can't do that. Their silent voices must be heard. The future suicides stopped years in advance. Understanding must be grown and spread. Spread understanding today, save a life tomorrow.

THE SPARK IN US ALL

We live in a world that is full of doubts and doubters but yet there is greatness achieved every day, throughout the world. There are people who ignore all of the reasons why not and just make it why. When everyone shouts "impossible!" they whisper back "watch me." We all have our battles, our demons, our fears but the truth is that those that suffer the most, have to fight even harder through the roadblocks. We all react differently to situations, yet so many of us follow the same path when any form of resistance presents itself. Those that do what others don't do are the ones that ripple the pond, etch a mark in history's line. I tell you now, if you want to leave your mark on this world, if you have any desire to set yourself apart from the rest, you can't do the same old thing. Sure, we have to know what has been done and worked in the past but that is only to build our knowledge for a base to build on. Learn from the past but mold your own path. Know what has been done but never fear to imagine and try what hasn't been done. Those that set new standards, find new light and bring new ideas into this world are forever remembered. Now, I am about to tell you the most important thing that you will ever need to know..... It is all on you. I shall say it again with more emphasis in case you take these words lightly. IT IS ALL ON YOU! You can NOT rely on anyone else to fight your fights, create your art or give you what you want from life. Don't get me wrong, it's fine to ask for help and receive assistance from others but it's YOUR actions that define you. We live in a cold and harsh world where people step over each other just to gain an inch and the ones you trust most would throw you under the bus just to feel better about themselves and their own lives. You must find the courage within yourself to do what you need to do for your soul's peace. I speak from a lifetime of severe depression, suicidal thoughts and a head full of bad memories and shit but here I am, living my life, writing every day and forging my own path. Yes, the haters and the ones that don't understand do get me down and do bring doubt into my heart but I do not let it stop me for long. I've read enough about the legends of history to know that the greatest ones have the most doubters. The ones that get called crazy are usually the ones that can think outside the box and bring amazing new things into this world. If you have ever felt like an outsider, a weirdo, a loser, just know that you are one of the special ones that is lucky enough to see the world a different way. A present wrapped in curses can often hold a glowing gift inside the darkness. Don't you ever feel bad about wanting it all to end, wanting to give up. When life is easy, risks are not often taken and rewards hardly satisfy. Those that put it all on the line for their dreams are the ones that win the biggest. Sure you can lose it all but if you have little to begin with, what have you to lose? You are the one and only you. Nobody is the exact same and nobody can look at the world the way you do. Embrace what sets you apart and use it to make your positive mark. I see you glowing, light fighting its way through the dark and it inspires me every day. So many people going through horrible times but the spark never dies. It may flicker and fade but it will always be there, burning at the core of your soul. Keep fighting your fight and walking your path. You are beautiful in your own special way and the only thing that can take that away from you is you giving up on it. Much love to you all and I hope you find that shiny spark inside you.

UNDERSTANDING FOR PROBLEMS DEVELOPED AS A CHILD

So many of us have been through this in one form or another. When a person deals with bad times at home and in the rest of the world in their childhood and also teen years to a lesser extent, these times before the mind is truly formed, deep lying issues can be formed that often wreak havoc with the way a person is able to deal with certain things in their adulthood. Too often these original issues come from the parents whom most of the time don't even realize the wounds they are inflicting. Parents fighting, arguing causing a child to be unable to deal with conflict of any type as an adult. Divorce making someone unable to trust commitment or love. There are so many ways we are affected when young. As children, we had no idea of what was going on in our heads when these problems formed and begun to affect us let alone be able to explain what we were feeling, going through. So many parents can't even afford to get real help for the children even when they realize they need it and some don't want to admit their child needs help as deep down they see it as a mark against their parenting to admit it. Problems that start at home spread out into life at school as any child that doesn't fit in or act like everyone else becomes a target, bullied and ridiculed just for being themselves, for having problems they are already struggling to deal with and don't even understand and likewise with problems at school coming home and growing. This in turn snowballs the mental struggles and self-issues and before you know it, all parts of someone's life are suffering and nobody at the school or at home can help or even try to help which I think is a reason all teachers should have at least some training in counselling as to spot problems early on and help the child deal with it, help the parents and child understand what is going on. There are too many youths being told they have to take medication and not enough being shown natural ways to deal like meditation. Without the proper help and changes where the problems are coming from, adulthood is reached and there is yet another adult whom doesn't have the tools to interact and function in society as the world expects them too so they are unfairly looked down upon even more, treated like an outcast, like they are not good enough or there is something deeply wrong with who they are, sometimes by the people whom gave them the issues that made them that way. We need so much more understanding for anyone whom is looked at by societies cruel standards as not fitting in or having problems. We need healthier and natural ways of helping deal with the problems and more acceptance of the people and the problems instead of judgement. So many of these people are struggling so hard just to deal with each day, just to keep fighting on in life. The weight they carry on their shoulders and soul so heavy and unbearable most of the time. It is a win just to get through a day, to be able to do things like go down the street or socialize with others.   To make normal relationships work like friendships and relationships can become impossible even with the right people. Show some love and understanding instead of judgement, please. It will ease the stress for so many trying to survive in a world they don't feel they can fit into.

THE BEAUTIFUL POWER INSIDE YOU

Although you may find the path you walk littered with jagged obstacles and haunting darkness, wounding pain and potholes, there is great shining light and incredible strength inside you that can burst glowing beams of light through any dark, lift you up with weightless wings above all hurdles. You may trip and stumble off the path but it is always there, never gone, waiting close by for you to find your feet upon it once again and steady your focus. If you find yourself lost, turning in circles and direction faded, you need only peer deep down inside yourself with open mind and willing heart to take a hold of your unique light and find your step back to where you need to be and ground is solid. The gift of life is such a fantastic miracle and you, you are life, you are a miracle, a beautiful glowing spark of creation that has unlimited potential inside you that flows from the great energy that enabled the beauty of life to exist. We are part of that powerful energy that makes all possible and in being a part of it, we share all its endless potential, beauty, power and light. Never look upon yourself as nothing or not good enough for you are a part of the almighty energy that flows through us all and the entire universe and all of existence with divine purpose and makes miracles possible. You just need to sync yourself with the energy, let your heart love, let your mind understand, let your soul grow. Learn what you can to make this possible and you can forge a path that brings you the truest joy, changes lives, achieves dreams and makes such a difference, be it to you or to many. You are life, you are a great miracle and you control your unwritten destiny. What falls upon the path that flows under your feet is out of control but your power to handle all that is in front of you is rooted in your soul, the atoms that make you what you are. Seek the truth of yourself and all that you truly can be for I swear on my own beating heart that you have more in you than you ever dreamed of knowing or imagined. Go forth, seek, embrace and discover. There is light you have yet to find.

THE BATTLE OF LIVING LIFE WITH MENTAL ILLNESS

I know I don't speak to the absolute truth of everyone's mental illness as so many of us suffer it differently but I am trying to spark light in those lives at the same time as bringing understanding to them. As much as growing understanding in the world for those that suffer from things like depression, bi polar, borderline personality disorder and other similar mental illnesses is important to me as there is still far too much stigma and ignorance in the world, I also really hope to spark something in sufferers like me that ignites even the tiniest of lights in their dark. Something they can use to clutch even a finger on outside of their life of struggle. So many people spout misunderstanding things like "just be happy" or "toughen up" and "get over it" "smile" when the chemical reactions and imbalance in our brains walls us off from being able to do such things at will, keeps us pinned down, drowning under the water of darkness, the weight of it all keeping us from breaking the surface, suffocating in the pressure of it all and having to use multiple times strength that most use just to get through every day. Depression pins someone down with unflinching force that gives them no inch, no air to breathe outside of their personal hell as much as they try to beat it, as hard as they try to grasp some freedom in their life to live like everyone else. Living with bi polar is different as it flips up and down between that crippling depression and manic highs but let me tell you this, when you spend a lifetime going up and down between those intense, insane highs and drowning, gutting, soul crushing lows, it messes with you so bad, hurts you like a normal person will never know. I have suffered from depression since I was a young child and only realized I have bi polar in my adult years so I know some of both. It isn't about going through bad things in life although many of us have, it is about the unbeatable troubles in our mind, heart and soul, the chemical reactions in our brain that can takes a lifetime of different meds to even come close to not quite helping so please show some understanding to those that suffer through this kind of life. It is not a mood we choose or a mental state we want to live with and although for some of us, there is ways in the world to counteract the chemical reactions, it is so very hard to find something that can have that effect. Please think next time you feel like telling someone to snap out of it because it might be so much more than them just being sad about something, they might be lifetime depression sufferers and suicidal.

YOU ARE, YOU CAN

There's a deep connection that flows through us all, a great energy with the power to heal all pains and spread so much light and love, yet there is still so much pain, hate and darkness in this beautiful world. Our minds and hearts have grown closed and cold where there is unlimited potential for almighty light and love if we can just learn to expand the way we think and feel. If we can look deeper into selves, others and the universe instead of having the restricted view we live with. Inside us all, right down from the very atoms we are made up of, the building blocks and energy of the universe and everything in it, there is incredible power, energy and potential. Potential for miraculous achievement, understanding, love, enlightenment and evolving of humanity. We as a species and each person can make a huge difference in the world, in other lives if we tap into the right energy and let it flow back out through us with the right frequency. Never underestimate just how much strength you have in you, how much you can achieve, the positive effect you can have on the world and other lives. You can get through any hardship, survive against the longest odds, win any struggle whether it be internal or in the world. If you can find a way to open mind to the truth of the universe, look deep into self and temporarily disconnect from the noise of society, you will find the way, the truth inside you that links us all with all that is and has ever been. You ARE love, light, life and powerful energy.

RELIGION AND SPIRITUALITY – CHANGING WORLD.

To begin with, I am not religious but I am spiritual. I have had religion in my life though as I was baptized and my grandmother used to take me to Anglican church. I was always extremely curious and excited about some of the stories from religion and wanted answers and proof which never came as religion is a faith based thing, not science. Some would say the same about spirituality but there is science to spirituality as well as faith. For me, spirituality is about our connection, at our very core of being, to everything that exists. The atoms that the universe is built upon and powered by which we are made up of as well and connects us with everything and all with us.

There is great energy, light and power in it all that flows through us and enables us to do great things, find peace in self, heal others just by focusing mind enough to tap into the right energy and send it out. Meditation is a big part of this as it allows us to remove all distraction of the materialistic world and center ourselves, delve into the metaphysical and spiritual world or plains. When we are able to look deep enough into self and find the energy, light and power of the universe in there, incredible things can be achieved. Illness of the body and mind can be beaten. We can transcend our physical body and step into the plain of light where some say God is. Some religion would say that meditation is the path to god. That going deep enough into self and mind and transcending body is how we can truly see and talk to him. The great Yogi, spiritual and religious leader Paramhansa Yogananda spoke of it often in his book 'Autobiography of a yogi' which teaches great love, kindness, spiritual and religious learnings as well as the power of meditation and yoga to change one's life and unleash previously unthought-of of potentials. I am not religious and I believe that the power of the universe is what many think God to be. The fact that so much hate, violence, bloodshed and bigotry is done in the name of religion makes me sick but I still think religion is a beautiful thing because so many good people, so many whom suffer find peace and meaning in it. It gives them warmth and light, takes away feeling alone in this world and gives purpose to a life lived with so much pain. I do find it disturbing that some religious people accuse atheists like me of being bad people because we have no god or religious beliefs to stop us being bad people but we don't need those things to be good people, to know what is right and wrong. It scares me that the fear of God might be the only thing stopping some religious people from being monsters, animals. Moral code and good beliefs shouldn't be reliant upon a God but should be based on just being good in self, knowing what is right in the world. We all make mistakes and have done things we are ashamed of or feel bad about. That is just part of life but we grow, we learn, we evolve as people and for the most part, we become better for it. There are so many similarities between religion and spirituality like the afterlife. Both believe in it, just in different forms. What some religion believes to be heaven, some spiritual believers believe is a higher plain of existence where our energy and soul rises up and can continue to evolve in goodness and keep rising up to even more enlightened stages of afterlife. Pretty similar huh. Religion prays, spiritual people meditate and both are connecting with the ultimate power be it god or the universe. I am grateful for the ways religion and spirituality encourage good in the world. The promotion of kindness, good energy, love and caring is so important and invaluable to humankind as we move forward as a species. I believe it is through spirituality, using meditation and encouraging the good energy beliefs that we can evolve to a utopian society. If all the bad energy in each and every one of us was swept away with the power of meditation than love, open minds, caring and unlocked potential would carry us with glowing wings to a better time, a better future for humankind where peace rules out greed and war. Love for fellow humans rids the world of famine. Evolved minds cure every disease and illness there is. A beautiful dream huh. It could be achieved if the essence and truest base meaning of religion and spirituality was embraced instead of all the different interpretations of what so many think they mean. We can change the world, evolve to something so much better if we go back to the base of love others, do good in its truest meaning with no interpretations that lead to doing bad for the sake of good. I know because of some countries in the world that this is a difficult thing to accomplish but we can start a movement that spreads. We can make sure the right energy grows strong in us, our lives, our countries and the world. It starts small but grows big and can change everything. Live and love.

THE FIGHT IN YOU

You've been rising up for so long now, giving it so much effort but lately it's just been getting too hard again, huh. You're wondering where the hell you're gonna summon the energy to go again, to keep fighting on and moving forward, like you're drained of all strength. Mind and body weary, run ragged but here is the thing. You DO have it in you, deep inside, that power, that potential to defy all odds and smash through those mental and physical blocks. You were created to be able to endure such terrible hardships and horrible tragedies and although it feels like you are at breaking point, like there is nothing left, there are almighty reserves of strength inside you. You are tapped into the flowing energy of the universe that connects us all and it can carry you forward, can keep your soul lit, fires burning and fuel yourself. I know that just the thought of going through the usual daily process looms over you after a while and the motivation hides from sight and feel. It can be so damn hard but you are such an incredible creation. You are magic in physical form, great power, unlimited potential and glowing energy all wrapped up together in the person that you are. Those roadblocks in front of you can be passed by like a giraffe goes by the blade of grass and you can keep going, can keep fighting and moving forward, pushing on past the point you thought you couldn't. Breathe, refocus, let your mind settle, your body loosen and step forward again with the purpose that screams for all to hear 'I WON'T BE BEAT!'

LETTER TO HOMOPHOBES

Now, I am only bi sexual but this still hits home hard with me because of how I have been treated in my life for being a bit different than most in the way I am. And because how I have seen others being treated and the gay friends, male and female I have had and still have whom have had to deal with such prejudice, ignorance and hate when we are all humans. When we are all one species yet some get treated worse than others which is a huge problem involving not just gay rights but minority rights and the right of pretty much anyone who isn't a straight white male with money. So to the point. To all the homophobic dudes out there. Imagine this. You have a son that looks just like you that you love with all of your heart and are so proud of. Would do anything to protect him. So one day when he is older, maybe a teenager, he discovers he prefers guys over girls. Other people start to find out because he trusted the wrong person or even just let his look linger on the wrong person for too long and now he is coming home in tears, beaten, bruised and bleeding because of how he is, something he has no control over and will be that way for the rest of his life. He doesn't want to tell you he got beat up and picked on by everyone because he is gay. He just wants to fit in but can't change the way he feels. He attempts to keep it from you so you won't be let down but you find out anyway. Now tell me, would you have the same opinion as before? Would your first thought be to make him feel like even more of an outcast and unloved in the very place that is meant to be safe and home or would you want to go crack some heads? Now remember that everyone is someone's son or daughter and they have to go through the same stuff as your son. Time for equality and understanding instead of dusty old opinions that aren't relevant anymore. This world needs more love, understanding and acceptance and less hate, ignorant thinking and cruelty. There are too many wars where man kill man and women kill women so why can't we have more of man loving man and woman loving woman? Why is it a bad thing for there to be love between two people, no matter their gender when there is so much hate, cruelty, cold and evil in this world that so desperately needs more love and warmth, compassion and understanding. May love guide your heart and all our hearts to a better world.

YOU'RE NOT ALONE

Although many of us walk this earth with hearts and souls that consistently feel alone, there are so many of us that feel the same, that ache in ways that you do and are torn in ways that you are and in knowing that, know that although you might be alone physically or emotionally, you are not alone spiritually and so many of us are sharing some of the pain that you share, feeling like you do and if we each send a little love and light back out into the universe for each other, we will all receive more back than we send out and although separated, we are not truly alone in this world for the unique pains we share connect us, no matter the distance. Let's try our hardest to give love to each other whenever we can, to spread warmth and keep each other from falling into a dark that can't be come back from.

CREATIVITY AND MENTAL UNHEALTH

I think it's safe to assume that most of us enjoy some movies, music, books and other creative arts that entertain us but for some, these things are the only reason we are still breathing, still here on this earth. The links between creativity and mental illness have become much more obvious as the years roll on. To think and see the world in different ways is a beautiful gift and also a heavy weight. I'm not afraid to admit that books got me through my childhood and music and movies got me through the older years. At this point in my life, writing creatively helps me a fair bit. Things weren't good at home when I was young and they were just as bad at school so hiding out in the library and losing myself in the worlds of R.L Stine, Stephen King, J.R.R Tolkien, Enid Blyton and many others was the perfect escape for me. All these new fascinating worlds, characters, emotions and ideas took me away from my depression and filled me with excitement and joy, like I was in there with them, all the bad stuff left behind in the real world. I loved creative writing for many years before I decided to take it seriously. Back then I didn't realize just how much writing little stories and song lyrics/poems helped me deal with a lot of the emotions and thoughts in my head that I couldn't control usually. The arts are an amazing way for us to use our creativity and also deal with not fitting in, in the world. A way to express thoughts and feelings that others normally can't understand but the creativity allows us to show them in other ways like painting, singing, acting, dancing, writing etc. We take some of the darkness out of ourselves with certain bits of our art and turn it into something that can touch the lives of others in a positive way. We spread some light on what it is really like to deal with these illnesses in a way that draws people in instead of scaring them away. The more we do this, the less alone others like us will feel and the more the world will understand and stop judging the sides of us we ourselves struggle to deal with. The feeling I get when I get writing done every day is like a sweet temporary release from some of the demons that haunt me. Like a natural anti-depressant that is much healthier than any pill. This is what the arts and creativity can do for us. It's an outlet for the bad stuff building up inside us. A therapy session that anyone around the world that can experience that art, can be a part of. Every time we create, we lift ourselves a little out of the dark and spark light in our life. Robin Williams was a severely depressed man but look how much joy and laughter he brought to the world, how many people with depression he spread some warmth to because he channelled what was different about him into his art instead of letting it dictate how he lived his life. "Great art comes from great pain." Can you imagine the colourless, lifeless world we would be living in if mental illness hadn't affected some of the greatest artists, musicians and writers through history? Beethoven, Van Gogh, Newton, Hemingway, Michelangelo, to name just a few. Then there's the more current crop like Kurt Cobaine, Heath Ledger, River Phoenix, David Wallace.

Nobody can say for sure but I'm willing to bet anything that without his

mental illness demons, Stephen King wouldn't have come up with so many

monsters and demons in his books or achieved anywhere near what he has.

The same illness that causes his brain to look at the world different and feel

out of place, allows him to write the way he does and have the ideas he does,

helps him to delve deep into dark places that his readers love so very much.

We can contribute so much to the world, create art like nobody has ever seen,

write stories that take you to worlds never imagined and write music that

touches places in your heart that you thought were numb forever. You can

find out things about yourself in the creativity of a wounded artist that you

never knew. Having dealt with mental illness most of my life and people

walking out of my life whom were close to me because they couldn't handle

me in my bad times, I have cursed it over and over and over, ached, wished,

begged with tears for a reprieve from it, just to be normal and not ruin

everything good in my life but then I write something from the heart, inspired

by my pain and others find comfort in the words. Some judge and hate "Just

harden up, everyone goes through stuff, most just get on with it without

complaining." That's a pretty popular saying from people that really don't

understand mental illnesses but it's worth that extra weight on the soul when

my words touch others that do understand and have similar issues to me. May creativity forever brighten your path.

TO THOSE WITHOUT LOVE

Here to those spending life alone or who spent valentine's day alone but wanted someone special to share it with. Times like this, time alone is going to make it all the more special, so much more powerful when you do find that right someone whom flips your lonely heart and shines joy upon it. That person that switches a light on in you that has never shone with such beautiful power before that point. That magic that your heart aches for is finding its way through life to be with you, to embrace you with all the warm loving energy you deserve and it will find you, will give your heart wings and sweep you off your feet to float among the bliss it brings. Keep on going, moving forward towards the time that powerful love enters your life and heart. It is out there, that special one, treading the path of life towards the point you two shall meet and embrace in something so powerful and beautiful all the pain from loneliness is forgotten.

WE CAN DO ANYTHING

In 2006 Mark Inglis, a paraplegic with no legs climbed mount Everest using prosthetic legs. If he could do that than what is stopping any of us from chasing after and achieving a dream that we only fantasize about? Nothing is impossible when you research and realize the depths of potential in each and every one of us. The true power we have inside that flows from the universe and the atoms that make up everything. All any goal needs is time, hard work, patience, determination and learning. If Oprah can be born into poverty as a black female in this world where white men hold so much power, be pregnant at 14 and go on to become a billionaire, one of the most respected people in the world and one of the most, if not the most influential woman in the world than why should your dream be thought of as too big? Why should your beginnings, surroundings and life stop your path becoming something so much bigger and better? Determination, will power, work ethic and never giving up took her so very far and it can you too. Imagine what you could do if you meditated regularly to open your mind even more to your true power and your connection with all that is. I know troubles in life make it hard, are such a distraction and can kill mood, energy and motivation but this is where you can truly stand out, by pushing through those things, not letting them stop your progress. I can't say don't be sad or stressed although meditation helps with those things but when you feel you can't or don't want to try, just keep making even the tiniest progress each day. Inch forward even just a little while in the depths and you will find yourself getting through the hard times quicker and will have progressed more towards your dreams and goals when you have made it past the down time. I don't know your specific trials and tribulations but I do know that ever since humankind started life, there has been great things done by countless numbers around the world. We have come from cave dwellers to the magnificent people of today with endless evolving inventions that would blow the minds of merely a generation or two ago, all because of people trying and trying, no matter the thousands of times they failed, they kept going and pushing and working, no matter what anyone said and how hard it was. Great feats of mind, body, soul, brain and heart are accomplished all the time but almost none with the right effort and time put in to make them happen. You are endless potential wrapped in human body and oh my, the things that can be done with these bodies we have. Truly incredible. You want that dream you fantasize about? Make it happen with all the work and time it takes and you will get there.

UNDERSTANDING INSTEAD OF JUDGING

There's so very many different pains in this life we lead and so many wounded souls that suffer from at least some of them. Yet fewer have harnessed the tools to deal with such pains, learned how to find the mighty power inside self, the glowing light sword to combat the dark demons. It's not expected for people to understand how it is for others but that is no excuse for judgement. We can always try to learn, understand as much as we can without personally experiencing the unique pains of others. We need more empathy and understanding, less ignorance and judgement. To take the time to listen and learn is such a beautiful thing in a world that can be so cold despite its glorious beauty. Never underestimate just how much it can mean to someone to open an ear instead of looking down a nose. To open your heart instead of peering from behind your inner walls.

WHY SOME PEOPLE REALLY LET DRUGS RUIN THEIR LIVES

I am not condoning drug use in anyway, just discussing it. Now, as much as it can ruin lives, change who people are and destroy goodness and families, I will not judge anyone for their drug use as nobody knows exactly what goes on in the mind of someone else and how hard things are for them. So many use drugs to escape the realities of a life they hate or feel they can't cope with. So many use it as a way to deal with devastating depressions, terrible tragedies, powerful pains to try and numb the feeling of it all, escape the crushing gravity of it all that drains them of all energy and light, pulls them down so far into darkness, cripples them. Yes, there are healthier ways to deal with such things like meditation, fitness and working out, religion and spirituality, even seeking professional help and I loathe to say medication as consuming addictions can grow from prescribed medicine too. Now I don't blame anyone for not finding a healthier way to deal with stuff instead of losing self in drugs as it is seen as the easy way, a quick escape and when someone is down so far, the lowest rung of the dangling ladder is what is grabbed for. I spent a few years using party drugs to escape reality and with hope I would overdose and die but they were never more than a weekend thing for me which is all I could afford back then in my rooftiling apprentice days. I spent the majority of my twenties high smoking weed though and I know it isn't much compared to harder drugs but it held my life back, my health, physically and mentally, my finances and it was an escape from having to deal, well a little anyway as it numbed the brain a bit as I would smoke far too much to try and shut my head up, would fry it for the sake of peace but I have thankfully been drug free for about a year now as I was meant to be moving to America to live with the girlfriend at the time and I wanted to be in better shape, physically and mentally so gave drugs up and although we broke up right before I was going to move over there, I haven't touched drugs since. I have known a fair few people whose lives have been destroyed by their drug use which was from them trying to escape pain and as tough as they looked to be, they just couldn't handle the harsh reality and needed that escape. I see friends with so much potential, so much beauty and spark that lose it all or at least bury it all under the effects of the drug use.

Friends have killed themselves because they just couldn't handle it any longer, needed the final escape or ended up needing so many drugs to numb the pain as tolerance to drug effects built up that they ended up just dropping dead from it. Of course there are others who just get into drugs for a bit of fun with friends and end up developing an addiction because their personality is built that way, have an addictive personality and they too find themselves ruining their life, losing good people that loved and cared about them, even losing their own life. Good honest people become criminals, starting by stealing from family and friends to pay for their addiction and spiralling into much worse crime, just to feed the need. So much of the drugs being used is mixed with dangerous chemicals and even poisons that end up frying peoples brains permanently and killing so many because it is all they can afford to get plus is easily made and very available these days, even in small country towns. I don't know how to stop this rampant problem as no matter how many drug shipments are stopped, drug dealers and smugglers locked up, new laws brought in and toughened up, there will always be cheap, low quality drugs being made and sold on the streets and out of homes in our countries, out cities, our country towns as there will always be a need for it.

Some things that can make a small difference but just might make the important difference in some lives are better spread of information to youth about the repercussions of it all, more and better available counselling services on a wide spread scale for the young and the old to help deal with problems before they grow to such a bad stage. I know so many don't want to talk to anyone, want to keep it to themselves and their friends they do the drugs with but there will be some that open up to the help of professional talking and that will be some lives saved. The same goes with family. I know most troubled teens, teens in general won't open up and talk to family but some will. It even needs to start at a much earlier age, the help and communication happening as there can be problems developed as a young kid, like depression and similar that might not be noticed or thought of as much until it has snowballed by the time they are older like did with me. There's not too much that can be done about keeping people from falling in with the wrong crowds. Yes, you can be tight as parents and keep kids as good as possible away from bad stuff and bad influences but that just makes some of the good ones want that lifestyle even more and fall into it deeper when they get freedom as get older. I have known a few really well brought up people whom were straight edge, goody goody whom once got some freedom of being old enough to do more of what they wanted, they fell into the drug life and completely lost themselves to it. I knew one person whom was so good, always reading books and listening to parents and she ended up dating a junkie and becoming one herself. I guess another problem solver that would help some is rehab being much cheaper and more of them available, something that is at least decently funded so people can get the proper help they deserve and teachings in there to make sure they don't relapse right back into the hole when they are back out in the world, doing it on their own again. Support networks are so important too although not everyone is so lucky as to have support that is understanding, loving, strong and reliable. Even some with all the help in the world, all the healthy alternatives, support, everything they need to survive and beat the battle can lose out and still end up taking their own life or losing self to drugs. But with continued improved knowledge, understanding and support avenues there can be more lives saved, even if only a few more each year which is more than worth it. Especially if you imagine that life being saved is someone you love or care about. Imagine if it is the future of one of your children being saved ahead of time. We all want to think, no I won't let it happen to me or my kids or someone I care about but better to have measures in place, better support and health systems for the good of all, just in case. It is a scary world yes, even more so for our kids to be growing up in but wrapping them in cotton wool to protect them can do more harm than good so it is up to us to make the world less dangerous for them, for all. We can do it. We can save lives.

LIGHT FROM CREATIVITY

We live in a world where although it is full of wondrous beauty and light, there is also so much pain and darkness. Things like music, books, dance, movies, all types of creativity can lift the soul, lighten the weight in heart and change someone's whole perspective and mood. They can turn unhappiness into joy, inspire such emotion, feeling and life among even the saddest of us with the right piece of creativity. How often have you felt your mood lift from a certain song or lost yourself in a book for hours upon hours, forgotten all the worries you were feeling. or been so touched by a movie you cried or felt electricity run through your whole body from these pieces of creativity that came from the mind of another. We have such incredible ability in us as humans to create things that can affect others so deeply, inspire, change lives, save souls. Let's have more encouragement of those whose dream it is, whose passion is to bring more of this creativity and beauty into the world for what would the world be without such amazing things.

WE THAT LIVE WITH THE DIFFERENT FORMS OF DEPRESSION

We that live with the different forms of depression are not lesser people because of it. We are not weak, not sad and can't 'just be happy'. To my fellow sufferers, don't ever let anyone make you feel like less than you are because they don't understand the draining battle you have to fight right through your life. I know that making it out of bed can be a victory in itself when other people are pushing for better jobs, buying houses, starting businesses. Yes, there are times when we do those things too and if others knew, if they really understood the amount of extra mental and physical effort and strain it took to do such things, the sheer force of will to use energy you don't even have, they would look at you different. I applaud all of you out there who suffer with the struggle in your own head. Those whose demons regularly beat them in battle. You whose lives feel empty of hope, drained of energy, missing light, love, purpose, you are the truly strong ones, as much as you may feel weak, you live lives that others take the ease of for granted. You still go on, still taking breath and doing just as much as others without the fuel in your tank to even be able to do it but you do, despite the demons, despite the judgement and lack of understanding. You are incredible people, so brave to keep fighting on, so courageous to face up to the world when it feels you don't even fit into it. If we can share our own knowledge of the pain to spread some light to others suffering through it, if we can grow understanding in the world about the truth of the struggles we endure then there will be some purpose in the pain, some more warmth in hearts and light in the dark. It won't be something we have to go through for no apparent reason. I know I have often broken down in tears, just wanting it to end, asking what's the point, why do I have to live with this, can't keep going on like this so I try and let others know they aren't alone in these battles, aren't the only ones with these unique pains. If we can make the world even just a little better for each other, imagine how many lives could be saved, how many might choose to keep breathing, keep going on when they reach that broken down in tears, just want it to end, moment.

SPIRITUALITY HEALS

Studying and practicing spirituality soothes my soul and eases the pain in my heart. I feel no need for religion or gods as my spirituality guides me with the greatest power there is. The power of the universe and all of its flowing connections that are a part of us all, tie us all together, the atoms that make up everything and are the energy of the universe and all in it. We are one with it and it with us which allows us (when the mind is awakened N open) to create any destiny we seek. We can achieve wonderful things with our powerful minds and the energy we are. The energy that is only temporarily carried in the physical body before reaching the next level of existence where we live as pure energy in a higher state of consciousness. When we learn to truly look inside ourselves and see and feel the energy of the universe there, we can use it to make incredible things happen, miracles by definition of most. Each and every one of us can use the energy that vibrates in everything to make fantastic things happen, realize our potential. Meditation is a key step for so many to start on this path while others are born with spiritual ability already peeking out from the surface of their subconsciousness. We are, you are more than just simply a human. You are divine potential, limitless power and glowing, pure vibrating energy. Don't ever feel like you are nothing or can do nothing for the greatest power there is runs through you, is a part of you as you are it, just waiting to be tapped into.

THAT FIGHT AFTER THE 100%

When you feel you are beaten by the weight of life. When you scrap for the tiniest bit of energy and come up empty handed. When you give your absolute all for nothing. When you reach and try and fight and work and scrap and scrimmage for that tiny bit of extra and you get nothing. This is when you must keep pushing forward with more spirit than ever before. When you must not let your light blow out. Must not let your heart weaken its resolve to reach what it wants. It feels okay to get and achieve what we want when it comes easy but it changes lives when you give your all and fight with all you have to get what you want and suffer through incredible pain to touch that glowing light at the end of the hard fought through tunnel.

ALL TOGETHER

May your light brighten the path of others and your dark let others know they aren't alone in theirs. Pain and joy, happiness and sorrow, they are all part of this beautiful mess we call life. The good and the bad make us who we are, shape a rounded perspective and full personality and view upon life. Don't look down upon those whom are weighed down by harder parts of life or those that are floating freely with little strain. We are all in this together, our energies all contributing to the beauty of the world, all sides of it, all just as much a part of the universal energy as the next. (Now when I talk of the darker sides, I do not mean evil people that commit evil acts. When I speak of darker side, I mean those of us whom suffer with depression and other such things that weigh heavy on our souls) We are all a part of this wonderful world, living side by side with each other, making our way along our paths, doing what we can and sometimes less than we can but always with heart beating. You, me, them, us, I, all of us are pieces of the beautiful puzzle that is life, energy, love and potential of this earth, this existence. Let's make it something that will be looked upon as good and right, warm and caring, loving and understanding. This is well within our capabilities and so much better for ourselves, our hearts, our souls, humankind and life in general.

TO THOSE JUDGED FOR THEIR BATTLE WITH DEPRESSION

You don't need to take more weight upon that depression than you already feel. Do not ever let anybody make you feel bad about how it cripples you, how it wreaks havoc with every day of your life, everything you try and do. Not many know just how crushing it can be, how unbearable, soul destroying, heart breaking, light stealing it can be, how it holds you under the surface, drowns you in your own dark while you kick and fight to gasp for breath that it won't let you breathe. So many say things like 'just be happy' or toughen up' or 'get over it' when we know that that is just not possible. So many spend their whole lives getting professional help and going through a never ending number of meds that give no help or ease to pain and no respite is ever found.

People grow tired of your depression and the way it affects you, if only they actually knew how tired of it all you were yourself, how you beg and cry and ache for some relief. How you have so many times where you just can't go on anymore and suicide feels like the only option you have. I just want you to know that you are not alone in your struggle as much as you may feel you are. There are many of us out here, so many that battle those 'demons' and lose the battle far more often than win. Some never feel a win, some find some light through the dark but still fight the battle daily and some are even lucky enough to find ways to heal the mind but we are all in this together. Don't ever let anyone make you feel bad for suffering the way you do. I often try to spark motivation and flick a switch in mind of others to try and get a chain reaction of positive chemical reactions going to counteract the depression but I know that only works on few yet it is worth it to try even if it only helps one. I know how annoying it can be to have someone tell you the way it works in your mind can be changed as people used to piss me off so much by underestimating just how hard it is and how it works but I never tell someone like us to just be happy I try to help them find ways to spark a different chemical reaction in brain to fight the 'demons.' I hope you all can find something in this life that brings you some light through the dark. My thoughts are with you.

CARPE DIEM

You control your glowing destiny. It's there to be grabbed with almighty strength and forged to the dream you seek, the dream that illuminates your beating heart. Reach out and take it, make it what you want, don't forsake it. Fate being out of control is the excuse of the afraid when we live in the world full of promise that most of us do. Roadblocks and pits can be leaped with faith powered strength which flows through you, comes from deep within, not from anyone else, just you and your eternal and internal power that comes from the very energy that makes up the universe. Waste not another breath before stepping towards the fate you want to make. You are your heaviest anchor and most powerful wings so start seizing the day, pushing forward before your time runs out. I believe in you, now you have to believe in you. You and only you make the fate, the future you want. You control whether you touch that beckoning light of what you seek from life or whether you simply gaze out at it with longing despair. Stand up and make the life you want, the future you want! Now is the time to really give that dream your all, you can do it!

DON'T LET THEM BRING YOU DOWN

Just because some people feel the need to bring you down for whatever reason, maybe their own issues or their perceived view of you, don't ever let a jaded opinion or flawed point of view make you feel bad about yourself. There isn't a person among us that is perfect. We all have at least some flaws that this at times cruel world gave us. Even the best of us have cracks but you are still a beautiful soul that doesn't deserve to be put down and most certainly doesn't deserve to be made to feel bad about the cracks life has given you. Don't ever forget that the rose that grew from concrete might have torn petals but the fact it made it through is testament to strength of self.

BE MORE THAN YOU HAVE SETTLED FOR

Here is the 100% truth of it, the honest, complete speech. Every single person on this earth can achieve greatness if they dedicate their lives to it, if they don't let anything get in the way of what they want to accomplish. Nobody was put on this earth to be nothing and do nothing. It is only what we limit ourselves to that truly holds us back. There are people living in war torn countries with nothing that grasp more than they thought they could so what is holding the rest of us back? Don't let the weight of your life pull you down. Do what you must and then do more. Be more than you have settled for. Be everything you have always wished and dreamed about. Be the glowing you that is hiding deep inside.

THOSE THAT SUFFER, KEEP FIGHTING ON

I don't have the horrific struggles of so many in the world but each day is such a draining battle to get through with these mental strains. So many of the days don't pass without tears of what haunts me from the past, the present and the pressures of the future. The 'demons' that poison my mind in their attempts to kill what is good in me and I fight oh so hard to use that to spark light and inspiration for more than myself. Although the battle brings me crashing to ground so much of the time, it also ignites white light from my heart and soul in hope of helping others and sharing the load we all carry, the weight that breaks us down, the world upon our shoulders that only we can feel and others scoff and mock. So here we stand or at least here we lay, still with one eye looking up with hope that someone else will understand and beam warmth onto our soul or at very least extend a hand to rise us up from our lowest point. Yet, we do not ask for help at all. We do this on our own. We march forward every day with all these burdens and put on poker face like we are rolling just like the rest. I feel you my fellow wounded warriors and just know you are not alone although in your life you may feel alone, we are a community across the world with shared scars and bleeding loving hearts. Every time you face the choice of giving up or continuing on and you make the decision to keep fighting on, your energy stays circulating among us all and helping the rest of us to continue. For if you quit and gave up, a little piece of all of us would die and the universal energy would weaken. Keep pushing on, keep fighting, keep moving forward with every ounce of strength your wounded heart can muster.

SPREAD LIGHT TO BRIGHTEN YOUR OWN

What you fear of tomorrow is born from the insecurities in self. Just know that you can survive any trouble, keep living through the hardest of problems and thrive despite any setbacks. We have time, we have breath and we have desire. Make what you can of your life and breed even more positivity into our world. It is what we make it, not what we want it but it can be what we want if we put in the effort to make it the way we want. I know for some of you it is near impossible to find hope and light, I feel you, I do. I spend much time in the depths of depression and darkness but I keep searching for ways to find light and have been lucky enough to have a passion for writing and meditation to give me focus, a heart that would rather bring light to others when I feel dark and the knowledge that every single human being has enormous potential for love and light if shown the right path. I tell you now, it's only the amazing feeling of being able to use my problems to help others that has helped me come to terms with the shit I go through. You can turn that dark into light through the hearts of others and your own deeds. We are all connected by unseen powers in the universe. The more light you bring to others, the less dark you shall have in your soul. However way you want to look at it, karma, religion, morals, self worth.. It's all about generating more good energy than bad. If you feel happy with your life but not truly happy with yourself, use your blessings to go grow some light in the darkness of someone else. If you feel hopeless, worthless and like nothing, use your experience of the dark to connect with others in the same type of situation. You will not feel so alone anymore and maybe even feel not so bad about your stuff while making others feel better about theirs. And if you are loving life, doing well, winning at this game, congrats and well done. But spare a thought for someone that could use a little extra help, someone that hasn't had the chances that you have or the strength inside to forge as far. Much love to every single one of you. We're all in this together, one world, a chance at something better.

THE SEEMINGLY IMPOSSIBLE BATTLE

I know you're hurting, I know it feels like it'll never end and the pain will drown you beneath the surface, like the dark will overwhelm you and steal all hope of light but you can beat it. I have dealt with some serious depression and it has always been the worst when I let it overwhelm me. I know it is so hard to imagine possible but you have to spark even the tiniest bit of light in yourself, reach for some hope in the future and it will have a chain reaction that slowly helps you fight back, find some joy in your life again. (I know that having mental illness can't just be switched off and turned to happy) I am saying that you have to will yourself to fight against it in any way you can and grow some strength in yourself, bit by bit until you aren't being demolished in the battle anymore. Whether it be with exercise, eating right, accomplishing a little something each day, anything to spark a better chemical reaction in brain against those already keeping you down. I myself am constantly up and down with severe highs and lows but it is so much better than the constant deep low I used to live in. I'm not telling you to be happy when you know you can't but I am saying you have to find something in this life that keeps you moving forward, gives you a reason to feel good about yourself when you do it. Much love to all those that are suffering in any way - rough time in life, mental illness, health problems, broken heart, death of close one, loss of job, failing studies, feeling alone in the world, anything that takes the light from your life. You can spark it again, I believe in you, in the power of the human mind and willpower and instinct to survive. Don't give up, okay. There is incredible power deep inside of you that you haven't even begun to tap into yet.

MEDITATION AND POTENTIAL OF SELF

Meditation is key to truth and peace in self and the energy we take in from and give back to the universe and the connections we share with it and all other life. To be more technical it is about metaphysics and the way we manipulate the atoms we are all made up of but spiritually it is about the power of your mind and soul to open up to the beauty of it all and become more in touch with it, more powerful and peaceful at the same time inside yourself and externally too. The energy is unlimited and when you realize your connection with it, you can flow with that same unlimited power and peace, achieve a state of mind that lets you live with love, kindness and light in the world where suffering people need it so very badly. Change in self first, find your peace and you'll be able to effect the lives of others in such positive ways.

THE CHOSEN PATH

There's a taunting echo that bounces rampantly around the minds of many that sometimes whispers, sometimes screams that there is no choice but what is laid out in front of you. That soulless voice tricks the mind into stumbling down a path that is oh so far from what the heart and soul yearn for yet it is walked none the less with the vigor that says it is not what is truly wanted and deep down you know that there is another path that beckons your honest desire. A road where although the potholes lay with deep bottom, the light flickers through the dark of the fog that covers said path. The light that glows with powerful hope as its battery. The light that can lift your jaded soul with soaring wings of heart's content. The path that your soul aches to walk is there for you to explore.

SHOW MORE UNDERSTANDING TO THOSE WITH MENTAL ILLNESS

If only everyone truly understood what it is like to have mental illnesses like manic depression/bipolar disorder/borderline personality disorder and depression in general, there would be a lot less judging in this world. Every moment of life can feel like a crushing weight, like we are tied down under water, far beneath the surface with the weight of the entire ocean upon us and just to keep living, surviving drains us of every ounce of energy we can muster. Like we are drowning so far down, surrounded by dark, no light in sight at all. The very act of breathing in oxygen for life is overpowered by a super vacuum inside us that sucks every bit of energy, hope, light, motivation and strength out. We don't want to be or sound negative. It's just the way things are and we try our hardest to keep moving forward and so many of us force fake smiles and keep it all to ourselves as much as we can. So many of us handle what we have to live with the best way we can and that's positive not negative. A negative thing about it is when people that don't understand it tell us to cheer up, stop being so negative, get over it, be happy like it is as simple as flicking a switch, like we want to be in the mental state we are. The positive side is that we are trying our hardest to still continue in this world like everyone else does, when just living like everyone else does is near impossible for us and fighting off suicidal thoughts sucks up so much of our daily energy. The simplest things in daily life can be so hard. The entire chemical reaction process in our brains is far more complicated than most and it is hell trying to deal with it, trying to be 'normal' or live like everyone else when our brains work so differently. We're giving it our best effort so please at least try to be understanding for those going through this lifelong battle. Show patience for someone who can't always react in the way you want or expect them to. Show love to someone who can't find love in themselves and never make someone feel even worse than they already do for the struggle they go through.

CHANGE THE WORLD

Trying to bring light, inspiration and understanding to those that suffer in the dark as well as achieving something great myself and touching the hearts of those already living in the light so that they may share some warmth. What can be done by some of us with incomplete power can be shared by all of us to create pure light and energy for all. If we all just share the load, the weight of others, then our own journey will be that much easier as well as theirs. If we spend less time judging and more time opening heart to taking real time to understand all sides and corners, the world will spin so much smoother and great energy will spread among us all. Great love and light will grow strength among us all and the world will change.

YOU HAVE THE STRENGTH INSIDE

You have such incredible potential for strength inside of, despite how life and pain and depression has weakened you and drained you of active strength. It is still inside of you, deep down, dormant while you suffer but you can feel the surge of its resistance again if you can find your way back to the bliss of deep meditation that will bring forth your power, let your strength and resolve rise again to aid you against those demons that wound you so deeply and terribly. You have made it this far and you CAN make it so much further, can fight back the troubles of mind and once again bask in joy and warmth. It IS in you to pull that strength back out of the depths of dark and ignite your life with light again.

BATTLE OF THE SEXES

We live in an age of new thoughts, understanding and growing equality but for some reason, society still pressures us to live up to stereotypes. "Men have to live without weakness" Looked down upon when any sensitivity is shown. "Women must be submissive to the man's world" Called bitches when they show strength of character. Men are forced into a corner of aggressive energy and made to keep all emotion held in until it bursts and women are pressured into playing a lesser role than what they could really be doing and given less respect for doing the same job as a man. Too many power struggles, no yard given. Not enough acceptance of anyone breaking the mold. Women, does it not drive you crazy to be called a bitch for standing up for your beliefs, showing you are equal and doing what men said you couldn't do? Men, does it not boil your blood to finally let your guard down, show you can be okay with exposing your weakness only to get told you are not a real man? I get it. It's only natural evolution that things take a long, long time to change but how long is too long? What can we do to shatter these out of date expectations? Is it not a sign of greater minds and intelligence to know that for a level society to exist, we must banish these "guidelines" for what we should be and let each person be comfortable and safe in their own unique personality? I spent almost ten years, on and off, working as a rooftiler, sweating and bleeding it out everyday around old school men, "hard" men that lived and died by old school standards. I picked up good traits from it, yeah. I learned the value of busting my ass and working hard to do what needed to be done but I always knew that wasn't how the full picture should be. How can we operate properly as a society when we're made to live in a way that isn't true to our personality? Why can't a female boss men without being called a bitch and being disrespected? Why can't a man admit weakness and cry without figuratively getting his nuts cut off? A woman in charge is still a female and a man in need of help is still a man. People will react negatively to change.. A man showing softer traits.. A woman showing harder traits.. Nobody likes to give any power away, give no inch and seize on any chance to get an upper hand over the other. Men, we need to stop making females feel bad about doing what we have done for ages, they can do it just as good, if not better and it does not make us any less of a person because a female can do it too We are all humans, all born equal. And women, you need to stop tearing men down for being what a lot of you complain about never finding. You want a good man but you destroy the ones that open their hearts to you. Isn't life and love a challenge enough without us making it harder than it needs to be? Can't we just work together to smooth the journey for us all? Love to you all and I hope these words save at least one relationship or friendship.